# The Flatulence Chronicles

# The Flatulence Chronicles

Matthew Petchinsky

# It's okay to fart

The Flatulence Chronicles: A Fart Journal for Self-Discovery
By: Matthew Petchinsky

**Introduction: Embracing the Logic Behind the Flatulence Chronicles**

When you first hear the word "fart," it might conjure up images of childish giggles and embarrassed glances. But let's set the record straight—there's absolutely nothing immature about keeping track of your flatulence. In fact, it can be a perfectly logical and insightful practice, rooted in medical reasoning. Your body is constantly giving you signals about what's going on inside, and paying attention to these signals can be a key to maintaining good health.

The **Flatulence Chronicles** is not just a quirky journal; it's a tool for self-awareness and well-being. Why keep track of your farts, you ask? Because they can provide vital information about your digestive health. Just as you would keep track of your diet, exercise, or sleep patterns, logging your farts can help identify potential triggers, patterns, or underlying medical issues. Whether it's certain foods, stress, or lifestyle habits causing changes in your body, flatulence is a natural occurrence that can often serve as a signpost to what might need attention in your overall health.

If you find yourself experiencing unusual discomfort, bloating, or changes in your flatulence patterns, this journal can become a valuable resource to share with your doctor. It might feel odd at first to discuss the specifics of your fart habits with a medical professional, but consider this: doctors deal with all aspects of bodily health, and understanding your digestive process is part of that. By tracking your flatulence, you are empowering yourself to notice how your body responds to different foods, stress levels, and activities. Over time, you might spot trends that can help pinpoint sensitivities, intolerances, or other medical issues that could be addressed early on.

So, welcome to the **Flatulence Chronicles**—a fun, lighthearted, yet genuinely helpful journey to understanding your body better. There is no shame in recording what your body naturally does. It's time to take your farts seriously and turn your gas into guidance!

Day 1:

**Date:** _____________________

**Time:** _____________________

**Location:** _____________________

**Mood Before the Fart: (Happy, Relaxed, Anxious, etc.)**

**Fart Details:**

**Sound:** (Silent, Soft, Loud, Explosive)

**Smell:** (Odorless, Mild, Strong, Overpowering)

**Duration:** (Quick, Prolonged, Series of Farts)

**Frequency:** (Single, Multiple in a row)

**Physical Sensations:**

**Before:** (Bloating, Pressure, Discomfort)

**After:** (Relief, Still Bloated, Discomfort)

**Diet Check:**
**Meals Prior:**

- ◦ Breakfast: _______________________
- ◦ Lunch: _______________________
- ◦ Dinner: _______________________
- ◦ Snacks: _______________________
- **Drinks:** (Water, Soda, Alcohol, etc.)


**Activity Check:**

- **Activities Before:** (Sitting, Walking, Exercise)


**Other Notes:**
(Anything unusual? Was it shared with others?)

Day 2:
**Date:** _______________________

**Time:** _______________________

**Location:** _______________________

**Mood Before the Fart: (Happy, Relaxed, Anxious, etc.)**

**Fart Details:**
**Sound:** (Silent, Soft, Loud, Explosive)


**Smell:** (Odorless, Mild, Strong, Overpowering)


**Duration:** (Quick, Prolonged, Series of Farts)


**Frequency:** (Single, Multiple in a row)


**Physical Sensations:**

**Before:** (Bloating, Pressure, Discomfort)


**After:** (Relief, Still Bloated, Discomfort)

## Diet Check:

- **Meals Prior:**
    - ◦ Breakfast: ___________________
    - ◦ Lunch: ___________________
    - ◦ Dinner: ___________________
    - ◦ Snacks: ___________________
- **Drinks:** (Water, Soda, Alcohol, etc.)

## Activity Check:

- **Activities Before:** (Sitting, Walking, Exercise)

## Other Notes:

(Anything unusual? Was it shared with others?)

Day 3:

**Date:** ______________________

**Time:** ______________________

**Location:** ______________________

**Mood Before the Fart: (Happy, Relaxed, Anxious, etc.)**

**Fart Details:**

**Sound:** (Silent, Soft, Loud, Explosive)

**Smell:** (Odorless, Mild, Strong, Overpowering)

**Duration:** (Quick, Prolonged, Series of Farts)

**Frequency:** (Single, Multiple in a row)

**Physical Sensations:**

**Before:** (Bloating, Pressure, Discomfort)

**After:** (Relief, Still Bloated, Discomfort)

**Diet Check:**

- **Meals Prior:**
    - Breakfast: ______________________
    - Lunch: ______________________
    - Dinner: ______________________

- ◦ Snacks: _____________________
  - **Drinks:** (Water, Soda, Alcohol, etc.)

**Activity Check:**

- **Activities Before:** (Sitting, Walking, Exercise)

**Other Notes:**

(Anything unusual? Was it shared with others?)

Day 4:

**Date:** _______________________

**Time:** _______________________

**Location:** _______________________

**Mood Before the Fart: (Happy, Relaxed, Anxious, etc.)**

**Fart Details:**

**Sound:** (Silent, Soft, Loud, Explosive)

**Smell:** (Odorless, Mild, Strong, Overpowering)

**Duration:** (Quick, Prolonged, Series of Farts)

**Frequency:** (Single, Multiple in a row)

**Physical Sensations:**

**Before:** (Bloating, Pressure, Discomfort)

**After:** (Relief, Still Bloated, Discomfort)

## Diet Check:

- **Meals Prior:**
    - Breakfast: _____________________
    - Lunch: _____________________
    - Dinner: _____________________
    - Snacks: _____________________
- **Drinks:** (Water, Soda, Alcohol, etc.)

## Activity Check:

- **Activities Before:** (Sitting, Walking, Exercise)

## Other Notes:

(Anything unusual? Was it shared with others?)

Day 5:
**Date:** ________________________
**Time:** ________________________
**Location:** ________________________
**Mood Before the Fart: (Happy, Relaxed, Anxious, etc.)**

**Fart Details:**
**Sound:** (Silent, Soft, Loud, Explosive)

**Smell:** (Odorless, Mild, Strong, Overpowering)

**Duration:** (Quick, Prolonged, Series of Farts)

**Frequency:** (Single, Multiple in a row)

**Physical Sensations:**
**Before:** (Bloating, Pressure, Discomfort)

**After:** (Relief, Still Bloated, Discomfort)

**Diet Check:**

- **Meals Prior:**
  - Breakfast: ________________________
  - Lunch: ________________________
  - Dinner: ________________________
  - Snacks: ________________________
- **Drinks:** (Water, Soda, Alcohol, etc.)

**Activity Check:**

**Activities Before:** (Sitting, Walking, Exercise)


**Other Notes:**
(Anything unusual? Was it shared with others?)

Day 6:
**Date:** _______________________

**Time:** _______________________

**Location:** _______________________

**Mood Before the Fart: (Happy, Relaxed, Anxious, etc.)**

**Fart Details:**
**Sound:** (Silent, Soft, Loud, Explosive)

**Smell:** (Odorless, Mild, Strong, Overpowering)

**Duration:** (Quick, Prolonged, Series of Farts)

**Frequency:** (Single, Multiple in a row)

**Physical Sensations:**
**Before:** (Bloating, Pressure, Discomfort)

**After:** (Relief, Still Bloated, Discomfort)

**Diet Check:**

- **Meals Prior:**
  - Breakfast: _______________________
  - Lunch: _______________________
  - Dinner: _______________________
  - Snacks: _______________________
- **Drinks:** (Water, Soda, Alcohol, etc.)

**Activity Check:**

- **Activities Before:** (Sitting, Walking, Exercise)

**Other Notes:**
(Anything unusual? Was it shared with others?)

Day 7:
**Date:** _______________________
**Time:** _______________________
**Location:** _______________________
**Mood Before the Fart: (Happy, Relaxed, Anxious, etc.)**

**Fart Details:**
**Sound:** (Silent, Soft, Loud, Explosive)

**Smell:** (Odorless, Mild, Strong, Overpowering)

**Duration:** (Quick, Prolonged, Series of Farts)

**Frequency:** (Single, Multiple in a row)

**Physical Sensations:**
**Before:** (Bloating, Pressure, Discomfort)

**After:** (Relief, Still Bloated, Discomfort)

**Diet Check:**

- **Meals Prior:**
    - Breakfast: _______________________
    - Lunch: _______________________
    - Dinner: _______________________
    - Snacks: _______________________
- **Drinks:** (Water, Soda, Alcohol, etc.)

**Activity Check:**

- **Activities Before:** (Sitting, Walking, Exercise)

**Other Notes:**
(Anything unusual? Was it shared with others?)

<u>**Week 1 review**</u>
**Week of:** _____________________________
**Total Number of Farts Logged:** _______________________________
**Most Common Time of Day:** ______________________________
**Most Common Location:** ______________________________
**Average Sound Level:**
(Silent, Soft, Loud, Explosive)


**Average Smell Intensity:**
(Odorless, Mild, Strong, Overpowering)


**Diet Observations:**

- Foods that increased flatulence: _____________________________
- Foods that reduced flatulence: _____________________________

**Activity Correlation:**

- Activities that seemed to increase frequency: _____________________
- Activities that seemed to decrease frequency: _____________________

**Notable Patterns or Changes:**

**Day 8:**
**Date:** _______________________
**Time:** _______________________
**Location:** _______________________
**Mood Before the Fart: (Happy, Relaxed, Anxious, etc.)**

**Fart Details:**
**Sound:** (Silent, Soft, Loud, Explosive)

**Smell:** (Odorless, Mild, Strong, Overpowering)

**Duration:** (Quick, Prolonged, Series of Farts)

**Frequency:** (Single, Multiple in a row)

**Physical Sensations:**
**Before:** (Bloating, Pressure, Discomfort)

**After:** (Relief, Still Bloated, Discomfort)

**Diet Check:**

- **Meals Prior:**
  - Breakfast: _______________________
  - Lunch: _______________________
  - Dinner: _______________________
  - Snacks: _______________________
- **Drinks:** (Water, Soda, Alcohol, etc.)


**Activity Check:**

• **Activities Before:** (Sitting, Walking, Exercise)

**Other Notes:**
(Anything unusual? Was it shared with others?)

**Day 9:**
Date: _______________________
Time: _______________________
Location: _______________________

**Mood Before the Fart: (Happy, Relaxed, Anxious, etc.)**

**Fart Details:**
**Sound:** (Silent, Soft, Loud, Explosive)

**Smell:** (Odorless, Mild, Strong, Overpowering)

**Duration:** (Quick, Prolonged, Series of Farts)

**Frequency:** (Single, Multiple in a row)

**Physical Sensations:**
**Before:** (Bloating, Pressure, Discomfort)

**After:** (Relief, Still Bloated, Discomfort)

**Diet Check:**

- **Meals Prior:**
  - Breakfast: __________________
  - Lunch: __________________
  - Dinner: __________________
  - Snacks: __________________
- **Drinks:** (Water, Soda, Alcohol, etc.)

**Activity Check:**

- **Activities Before:** (Sitting, Walking, Exercise)

**Other Notes:**
(Anything unusual? Was it shared with others?)

**Day 10:**
**Date:** _______________________
**Time:** _______________________
**Location:** _______________________
**Mood Before the Fart: (Happy, Relaxed, Anxious, etc.)**

**Fart Details:**
**Sound:** (Silent, Soft, Loud, Explosive)

**Smell:** (Odorless, Mild, Strong, Overpowering)

**Duration:** (Quick, Prolonged, Series of Farts)

**Frequency:** (Single, Multiple in a row)

**Physical Sensations:**
**Before:** (Bloating, Pressure, Discomfort)

**After:** (Relief, Still Bloated, Discomfort)

**Diet Check:**

- **Meals Prior:**
    - Breakfast: _______________________
    - Lunch: _______________________
    - Dinner: _______________________
    - Snacks: _______________________
- **Drinks:** (Water, Soda, Alcohol, etc.)

**Activity Check:**

- **Activities Before:** (Sitting, Walking, Exercise)

**Other Notes:**
(Anything unusual? Was it shared with others?)

Day 11:

**Date:** ______________________

**Time:** ______________________

**Location:** ______________________

**Mood Before the Fart: (Happy, Relaxed, Anxious, etc.)**

**Fart Details:**

**Sound:** (Silent, Soft, Loud, Explosive)

**Smell:** (Odorless, Mild, Strong, Overpowering)

**Duration:** (Quick, Prolonged, Series of Farts)

**Frequency:** (Single, Multiple in a row)

**Physical Sensations:**

**Before:** (Bloating, Pressure, Discomfort)

**After:** (Relief, Still Bloated, Discomfort)

**Diet Check:**

- **Meals Prior:**
    - Breakfast: ______________________
    - Lunch: ______________________
    - Dinner: ______________________
    - Snacks: ______________________
- **Drinks:** (Water, Soda, Alcohol, etc.)

**Activity Check:**

- **Activities Before:** (Sitting, Walking, Exercise)

**Other Notes:**
(Anything unusual? Was it shared with others?)

Day 12:

**Date:** ___________________________

**Time:** ___________________________

**Location:** ___________________________

**Mood Before the Fart: (Happy, Relaxed, Anxious, etc.)**

**Fart Details:**

**Sound:** (Silent, Soft, Loud, Explosive)

**Smell:** (Odorless, Mild, Strong, Overpowering)

**Duration:** (Quick, Prolonged, Series of Farts)

**Frequency:** (Single, Multiple in a row)

**Physical Sensations:**

**Before:** (Bloating, Pressure, Discomfort)

**After:** (Relief, Still Bloated, Discomfort)

**Diet Check:**

- **Meals Prior:**
    - Breakfast: ___________________
    - Lunch: ___________________
    - Dinner: ___________________
    - Snacks: ___________________
- **Drinks:** (Water, Soda, Alcohol, etc.)

**Activity Check:**

- **Activities Before:** (Sitting, Walking, Exercise)

**Other Notes:**
(Anything unusual? Was it shared with others?)

Day 13:

**Date:** ___________________________

**Time:** ___________________________

**Location:** ___________________________

**Mood Before the Fart: (Happy, Relaxed, Anxious, etc.)**

**Fart Details:**

**Sound:** (Silent, Soft, Loud, Explosive)

**Smell:** (Odorless, Mild, Strong, Overpowering)

**Duration:** (Quick, Prolonged, Series of Farts)

**Frequency:** (Single, Multiple in a row)

**Physical Sensations:**

**Before:** (Bloating, Pressure, Discomfort)

**After:** (Relief, Still Bloated, Discomfort)

**Diet Check:**

- **Meals Prior:**
    - Breakfast: ___________________
    - Lunch: ___________________
    - Dinner: ___________________
    - Snacks: ___________________
- **Drinks:** (Water, Soda, Alcohol, etc.)

**Activity Check:**

- **Activities Before:** (Sitting, Walking, Exercise)

**Other Notes:**
(Anything unusual? Was it shared with others?)

**Day 14:**
**Date:** ___________________________
**Time:** ___________________________
**Location:** ___________________________
**Mood Before the Fart: (Happy, Relaxed, Anxious, etc.)**

**Fart Details:**
**Sound:** (Silent, Soft, Loud, Explosive)

**Smell:** (Odorless, Mild, Strong, Overpowering)

**Duration:** (Quick, Prolonged, Series of Farts)

**Frequency:** (Single, Multiple in a row)

**Physical Sensations:**
**Before:** (Bloating, Pressure, Discomfort)

**After:** (Relief, Still Bloated, Discomfort)

**Diet Check:**

- **Meals Prior:**
    - Breakfast: ___________________________
    - Lunch: ___________________________
    - Dinner: ___________________________
    - Snacks: ___________________________
- **Drinks:** (Water, Soda, Alcohol, etc.)

**Activity Check:**

- **Activities Before:** (Sitting, Walking, Exercise)

**Other Notes:**
(Anything unusual? Was it shared with others?)

<u>**Week 2 Review**</u>
**Week of:** ___________________________
**Total Number of Farts Logged:** ___________________________
**Most Common Time of Day:** ___________________________
**Most Common Location:** ___________________________
**Average Sound Level:**
(Silent, Soft, Loud, Explosive)

**Average Smell Intensity:**
(Odorless, Mild, Strong, Overpowering)

**Diet Observations:**

- Foods that increased flatulence: ___________________________
- Foods that reduced flatulence: ___________________________

**Activity Correlation:**

- Activities that seemed to increase frequency:
  ___________________________
- Activities that seemed to decrease frequency:
  ___________________________

**Notable Patterns or Changes:**

Day 15:

**Date:** ___________________________

**Time:** ___________________________

**Location:** ___________________________

**Mood Before the Fart: (Happy, Relaxed, Anxious, etc.)**

**Fart Details:**

**Sound:** (Silent, Soft, Loud, Explosive)

**Smell:** (Odorless, Mild, Strong, Overpowering)

**Duration:** (Quick, Prolonged, Series of Farts)

**Frequency:** (Single, Multiple in a row)

**Physical Sensations:**

**Before:** (Bloating, Pressure, Discomfort)

**After:** (Relief, Still Bloated, Discomfort)

**Diet Check:**

- **Meals Prior:**
  - Breakfast: ___________________
  - Lunch: ___________________
  - Dinner: ___________________
  - Snacks: ___________________
- **Drinks:** (Water, Soda, Alcohol, etc.)

**Activity Check:**

• **Activities Before:** (Sitting, Walking, Exercise)

**Other Notes:**
(Anything unusual? Was it shared with others?)

Day 16:
**Date:** _______________________
**Time:** _______________________
**Location:** _______________________
**Mood Before the Fart: (Happy, Relaxed, Anxious, etc.)**

**Fart Details:**
**Sound:** (Silent, Soft, Loud, Explosive)

**Smell:** (Odorless, Mild, Strong, Overpowering)

**Duration:** (Quick, Prolonged, Series of Farts)

**Frequency:** (Single, Multiple in a row)

**Physical Sensations:**
**Before:** (Bloating, Pressure, Discomfort)

**After:** (Relief, Still Bloated, Discomfort)

**Diet Check:**

- **Meals Prior:**
    - Breakfast: _______________________
    - Lunch: _______________________
    - Dinner: _______________________
    - Snacks: _______________________
- **Drinks:** (Water, Soda, Alcohol, etc.)

**Activity Check:**

- **Activities Before:** (Sitting, Walking, Exercise)

**Other Notes:**
(Anything unusual? Was it shared with others?)

Day 17:

**Date:** ______________________

**Time:** ______________________

**Location:** ______________________

**Mood Before the Fart: (Happy, Relaxed, Anxious, etc.)**

**Fart Details:**

**Sound:** (Silent, Soft, Loud, Explosive)

**Smell:** (Odorless, Mild, Strong, Overpowering)

**Duration:** (Quick, Prolonged, Series of Farts)

**Frequency:** (Single, Multiple in a row)

**Physical Sensations:**

**Before:** (Bloating, Pressure, Discomfort)

**After:** (Relief, Still Bloated, Discomfort)

**Diet Check:**

- **Meals Prior:**
    - Breakfast: ______________________
    - Lunch: ______________________
    - Dinner: ______________________
    - Snacks: ______________________
- **Drinks:** (Water, Soda, Alcohol, etc.)

**Activity Check:**

- **Activities Before:** (Sitting, Walking, Exercise)

**Other Notes:**
(Anything unusual? Was it shared with others?)

Day 18:
**Date:** ______________________
**Time:** ______________________
**Location:** ______________________
**Mood Before the Fart: (Happy, Relaxed, Anxious, etc.)**

**Fart Details:**
**Sound:** (Silent, Soft, Loud, Explosive)

**Smell:** (Odorless, Mild, Strong, Overpowering)

**Duration:** (Quick, Prolonged, Series of Farts)

**Frequency:** (Single, Multiple in a row)

**Physical Sensations:**
**Before:** (Bloating, Pressure, Discomfort)

**After:** (Relief, Still Bloated, Discomfort)

**Diet Check:**

- **Meals Prior:**
    - Breakfast: ______________________
    - Lunch: ______________________
    - Dinner: ______________________
    - Snacks: ______________________
- **Drinks:** (Water, Soda, Alcohol, etc.)

**Activity Check:**

• **Activities Before:** (Sitting, Walking, Exercise)

**Other Notes:**
(Anything unusual? Was it shared with others?)

Day 19:
**Date:** ______________________
**Time:** ______________________
**Location:** ______________________
**Mood Before the Fart: (Happy, Relaxed, Anxious, etc.)**

**Fart Details:**
**Sound:** (Silent, Soft, Loud, Explosive)

**Smell:** (Odorless, Mild, Strong, Overpowering)

**Duration:** (Quick, Prolonged, Series of Farts)

**Frequency:** (Single, Multiple in a row)

**Physical Sensations:**
**Before:** (Bloating, Pressure, Discomfort)

**After:** (Relief, Still Bloated, Discomfort)

**Diet Check:**

- **Meals Prior:**
    - Breakfast: ______________________
    - Lunch: ______________________
    - Dinner: ______________________
    - Snacks: ______________________
- **Drinks:** (Water, Soda, Alcohol, etc.)

**Activity Check:**

- **Activities Before:** (Sitting, Walking, Exercise)

**Other Notes:**
(Anything unusual? Was it shared with others?)

Day 20:

**Date:** _______________________

**Time:** _______________________

**Location:** _______________________

**Mood Before the Fart: (Happy, Relaxed, Anxious, etc.)**

**Fart Details:**

**Sound:** (Silent, Soft, Loud, Explosive)

**Smell:** (Odorless, Mild, Strong, Overpowering)

**Duration:** (Quick, Prolonged, Series of Farts)

**Frequency:** (Single, Multiple in a row)

**Physical Sensations:**

**Before:** (Bloating, Pressure, Discomfort)

**After:** (Relief, Still Bloated, Discomfort)

**Diet Check:**

- **Meals Prior:**
    - Breakfast: _______________________
    - Lunch: _______________________
    - Dinner: _______________________
    - Snacks: _______________________
- **Drinks:** (Water, Soda, Alcohol, etc.)

**Activity Check:**

- **Activities Before:** (Sitting, Walking, Exercise)

**Other Notes:**
(Anything unusual? Was it shared with others?)

**Day 21**
**Date:** _______________________
**Time:** _______________________
**Location:** _______________________
**Mood Before the Fart: (Happy, Relaxed, Anxious, etc.)**

**Fart Details:**
**Sound:** (Silent, Soft, Loud, Explosive)

**Smell:** (Odorless, Mild, Strong, Overpowering)

**Duration:** (Quick, Prolonged, Series of Farts)

**Frequency:** (Single, Multiple in a row)

**Physical Sensations:**
**Before:** (Bloating, Pressure, Discomfort)

**After:** (Relief, Still Bloated, Discomfort)

**Diet Check:**

- **Meals Prior:**
    - Breakfast: _______________________
    - Lunch: _______________________
    - Dinner: _______________________
    - Snacks: _______________________
- **Drinks:** (Water, Soda, Alcohol, etc.)

**Activity Check:**

* **Activities Before:** (Sitting, Walking, Exercise)

**Other Notes:**
(Anything unusual? Was it shared with others?)

<u>**Week 3 Review**</u>
**Week of:** _______________________
**Total Number of Farts Logged:** _______________________
**Most Common Time of Day:** _______________________
**Most Common Location:** _______________________
**Average Sound Level:**
(Silent, Soft, Loud, Explosive)

**Average Smell Intensity:**
(Odorless, Mild, Strong, Overpowering)

**Diet Observations:**

- Foods that increased flatulence: _______________________
- Foods that reduced flatulence: _______________________

**Activity Correlation:**

- Activities that seemed to increase frequency:
  _______________________
- Activities that seemed to decrease frequency:
  _______________________

**Notable Patterns or Changes:**

Day 22
**Date:** _______________________
**Time:** _______________________
**Location:** _______________________
**Mood Before the Fart: (Happy, Relaxed, Anxious, etc.)**

**Fart Details:**
**Sound:** (Silent, Soft, Loud, Explosive)

**Smell:** (Odorless, Mild, Strong, Overpowering)

**Duration:** (Quick, Prolonged, Series of Farts)

**Frequency:** (Single, Multiple in a row)

**Physical Sensations:**
**Before:** (Bloating, Pressure, Discomfort)

**After:** (Relief, Still Bloated, Discomfort)

**Diet Check:**

- **Meals Prior:**
    - Breakfast: _______________________
    - Lunch: _______________________
    - Dinner: _______________________
    - Snacks: _______________________
- **Drinks:** (Water, Soda, Alcohol, etc.)

**Activity Check:**

- **Activities Before:** (Sitting, Walking, Exercise)

**Other Notes:**
(Anything unusual? Was it shared with others?)

Day 23
**Date:** ___________________________
**Time:** ___________________________
**Location:** ___________________________
**Mood Before the Fart: (Happy, Relaxed, Anxious, etc.)**

**Fart Details:**
**Sound:** (Silent, Soft, Loud, Explosive)

**Smell:** (Odorless, Mild, Strong, Overpowering)

**Duration:** (Quick, Prolonged, Series of Farts)

**Frequency:** (Single, Multiple in a row)

**Physical Sensations:**
**Before:** (Bloating, Pressure, Discomfort)

**After:** (Relief, Still Bloated, Discomfort)

**Diet Check:**

- **Meals Prior:**
    - Breakfast: ___________________
    - Lunch: ___________________
    - Dinner: ___________________
    - Snacks: ___________________
- **Drinks:** (Water, Soda, Alcohol, etc.)

**Activity Check:**

- **Activities Before:** (Sitting, Walking, Exercise)

**Other Notes:**
(Anything unusual? Was it shared with others?

Day 24
**Date:** ___________________________
**Time:** ___________________________
**Location:** ___________________________
**Mood Before the Fart: (Happy, Relaxed, Anxious, etc.)**

**Fart Details:**
**Sound:** (Silent, Soft, Loud, Explosive)

**Smell:** (Odorless, Mild, Strong, Overpowering)

**Duration:** (Quick, Prolonged, Series of Farts)

**Frequency:** (Single, Multiple in a row)

**Physical Sensations:**
**Before:** (Bloating, Pressure, Discomfort)

**After:** (Relief, Still Bloated, Discomfort)

**Diet Check:**

- **Meals Prior:**
    - Breakfast: ___________________________
    - Lunch: ___________________________
    - Dinner: ___________________________
    - Snacks: ___________________________
- **Drinks:** (Water, Soda, Alcohol, etc.)

**Activity Check:**

- **Activities Before:** (Sitting, Walking, Exercise)

**Other Notes:**
(Anything unusual? Was it shared with others?)

Day 25
**Date:** _______________________
**Time:** _______________________
**Location:** _______________________
**Mood Before the Fart: (Happy, Relaxed, Anxious, etc.)**

**Fart Details:**
**Sound:** (Silent, Soft, Loud, Explosive)

**Smell:** (Odorless, Mild, Strong, Overpowering)

**Duration:** (Quick, Prolonged, Series of Farts)

**Frequency:** (Single, Multiple in a row)

**Physical Sensations:**
**Before:** (Bloating, Pressure, Discomfort)

**After:** (Relief, Still Bloated, Discomfort)

**Diet Check:**

- **Meals Prior:**
    - Breakfast: _______________________
    - Lunch: _______________________
    - Dinner: _______________________
    - Snacks: _______________________
- **Drinks:** (Water, Soda, Alcohol, etc.)

**Activity Check:**

- **Activities Before:** (Sitting, Walking, Exercise)

**Other Notes:**
(Anything unusual? Was it shared with others?)

Day 26
**Date:** ______________________
**Time:** ______________________
**Location:** ______________________
**Mood Before the Fart: (Happy, Relaxed, Anxious, etc.)**

**Fart Details:**
**Sound:** (Silent, Soft, Loud, Explosive)

**Smell:** (Odorless, Mild, Strong, Overpowering)

**Duration:** (Quick, Prolonged, Series of Farts)

**Frequency:** (Single, Multiple in a row)

**Physical Sensations:**
**Before:** (Bloating, Pressure, Discomfort)

**After:** (Relief, Still Bloated, Discomfort)

**Diet Check:**

- **Meals Prior:**
    - Breakfast: ______________________
    - Lunch: ______________________
    - Dinner: ______________________
    - Snacks: ______________________
- **Drinks:** (Water, Soda, Alcohol, etc.)

**Activity Check:**

- **Activities Before:** (Sitting, Walking, Exercise)

**Other Notes:**
(Anything unusual? Was it shared with others?)

Day 27

**Date:** _______________________

**Time:** _______________________

**Location:** _______________________

**Mood Before the Fart: (Happy, Relaxed, Anxious, etc.)**

**Fart Details:**

**Sound:** (Silent, Soft, Loud, Explosive)

**Smell:** (Odorless, Mild, Strong, Overpowering)

**Duration:** (Quick, Prolonged, Series of Farts)

**Frequency:** (Single, Multiple in a row)

**Physical Sensations:**

**Before:** (Bloating, Pressure, Discomfort)

**After:** (Relief, Still Bloated, Discomfort)

**Diet Check:**

- **Meals Prior:**
    - Breakfast: _______________________
    - Lunch: _______________________
    - Dinner: _______________________
    - Snacks: _______________________
- **Drinks:** (Water, Soda, Alcohol, etc.)

**Activity Check:**

- **Activities Before:** (Sitting, Walking, Exercise)

**Other Notes:**
(Anything unusual? Was it shared with others?)

Day 28

**Date:** _______________________

**Time:** _______________________

**Location:** _______________________

**Mood Before the Fart: (Happy, Relaxed, Anxious, etc.)**

**Fart Details:**

**Sound:** (Silent, Soft, Loud, Explosive)

**Smell:** (Odorless, Mild, Strong, Overpowering)

**Duration:** (Quick, Prolonged, Series of Farts)

**Frequency:** (Single, Multiple in a row)

**Physical Sensations:**

**Before:** (Bloating, Pressure, Discomfort)

**After:** (Relief, Still Bloated, Discomfort)

**Diet Check:**

- **Meals Prior:**
    - Breakfast: _______________________
    - Lunch: _______________________
    - Dinner: _______________________
    - Snacks: _______________________
- **Drinks:** (Water, Soda, Alcohol, etc.)

## Activity Check:

- **Activities Before:** (Sitting, Walking, Exercise)

## Other Notes:
(Anything unusual? Was it shared with others?)

<u>**WEEK 4 Review**</u>
**Week of:** ___________________________
**Total Number of Farts Logged:** ___________________________
**Most Common Time of Day:** ___________________________
**Most Common Location:** ___________________________
**Average Sound Level:**
(Silent, Soft, Loud, Explosive)

**Average Smell Intensity:**
(Odorless, Mild, Strong, Overpowering)

**Diet Observations:**

- Foods that increased flatulence: ___________________________
- Foods that reduced flatulence: ___________________________

**Activity Correlation:**

- Activities that seemed to increase frequency: ___________________________
- Activities that seemed to decrease frequency: ___________________________

**Notable Patterns or Changes:**

Day 29
**Date:** ___________________________
**Time:** ___________________________
**Location:** ___________________________
**Mood Before the Fart: (Happy, Relaxed, Anxious, etc.)**

**Fart Details:**
**Sound:** (Silent, Soft, Loud, Explosive)

**Smell:** (Odorless, Mild, Strong, Overpowering)

**Duration:** (Quick, Prolonged, Series of Farts)

**Frequency:** (Single, Multiple in a row)

**Physical Sensations:**
**Before:** (Bloating, Pressure, Discomfort)

**After:** (Relief, Still Bloated, Discomfort)

**Diet Check:**

- **Meals Prior:**
    - Breakfast: ___________________________
    - Lunch: ___________________________
    - Dinner: ___________________________
    - Snacks: ___________________________
- **Drinks:** (Water, Soda, Alcohol, etc.)

**Activity Check:**

- **Activities Before:** (Sitting, Walking, Exercise)

**Other Notes:**
(Anything unusual? Was it shared with others?)

Day 30
**Date:** _________________________
**Time:** _________________________
**Location:** _________________________
**Mood Before the Fart: (Happy, Relaxed, Anxious, etc.)**

**Fart Details:**
**Sound:** (Silent, Soft, Loud, Explosive)

**Smell:** (Odorless, Mild, Strong, Overpowering)

**Duration:** (Quick, Prolonged, Series of Farts)

**Frequency:** (Single, Multiple in a row)

**Physical Sensations:**
**Before:** (Bloating, Pressure, Discomfort)

**After:** (Relief, Still Bloated, Discomfort)

**Diet Check:**

- **Meals Prior:**
    - Breakfast: _________________________
    - Lunch: _________________________
    - Dinner: _________________________
    - Snacks: _________________________
- **Drinks:** (Water, Soda, Alcohol, etc.)

**Activity Check:**

- **Activities Before:** (Sitting, Walking, Exercise)

**Other Notes:**
(Anything unusual? Was it shared with others?)

Day 31

**Date:** ______________________

**Time:** ______________________

**Location:** ______________________

**Mood Before the Fart: (Happy, Relaxed, Anxious, etc.)**

**Fart Details:**

**Sound:** (Silent, Soft, Loud, Explosive)

**Smell:** (Odorless, Mild, Strong, Overpowering)

**Duration:** (Quick, Prolonged, Series of Farts)

**Frequency:** (Single, Multiple in a row)

**Physical Sensations:**

**Before:** (Bloating, Pressure, Discomfort)

**After:** (Relief, Still Bloated, Discomfort)

**Diet Check:**

- **Meals Prior:**
    - Breakfast: ______________________
    - Lunch: ______________________
    - Dinner: ______________________
    - Snacks: ______________________
- **Drinks:** (Water, Soda, Alcohol, etc.)

**Activity Check:**

- **Activities Before:** (Sitting, Walking, Exercise)

**Other Notes:**
(Anything unusual? Was it shared with others?)

**<u>Monthly Review</u>**

**Month of:** _______________________

**Total Number of Farts Logged:** _______________________

**Most Common Weekly Pattern:**

(E.g., More farts on weekdays vs. weekends)

**Dietary Impact Summary:**

- **Top Flatulence-Inducing Foods:** _______________________
- **Foods that Alleviated Flatulence:** _______________________

**Lifestyle Observations:**

- Correlation between stress and flatulence: _______________________

- Correlation between physical activity and flatulence: _______________________

**Significant Changes Noticed This Month:**

(Changes in diet, lifestyle, or health)

**Goals for Next Month:**

(E.g., Adjust diet, increase water intake, change exercise routine)

<u>Message from the Author:</u>

I hope you enjoyed this book, I love astrology and knew there was not a book such as this out on the shelf. I love metaphysical items as well. Please check out my other books:

-Life of Government Benefits

-My life of Hell

-My life with Hydrocephalus

-Red Sky

-World Domination:Woman's rule

-World Domination:Woman's Rule 2: The War

-Life and Banishment of Apophis: book 1

-The Kidney Friendly Diet

-The Ultimate Hemp Cookbook

-Creating a Dispensary(legally)

-Cleanliness throughout life: the importance of showering from childhood to adulthood.

-Strong Roots: The Risks of Overcoddling children

-Hemp Horoscopes: Cosmic Insights and Earthly Healing

- Celestial Hemp Navigating the Zodiac: Through the Green Cosmos

-Astrological Hemp: Aligning The Stars with Earth's Ancient Herb

-The Astrological Guide to Hemp: Stars, Signs, and Sacred Leaves

-Green Growth: Innovative Marketing Strategies for your Hemp Products and Dispensary

-Cosmic Cannabis

-Astrological Munchies

-Henry The Hemp

-Zodiacal Roots: The Astrological Soul Of Hemp

- **Green Constellations: Intersection of Hemp and Zodiac**

-Hemp in The Houses: An astrological Adventure Through The Cannabis Galaxy

-Galactic Ganja Guide

Heavenly Hemp

Zodiac Leaves

Doctor Who Astrology

Cannastrology

Stellar Satvias and Cosmic Indicas

Celestial Cannabis: A Zodiac Journey

AstroHerbology: The Sky and The Soil: Volume 1

AstroHerbology:Celestial Cannabis:Volume 2

Cosmic Cannabis Cultivation

The Starry Guide to Herbal Harmony: Volume 1

The Starry Guide to Herbal Harmony: Cannabis Universe: Volume 2

Yugioh Astrology: Astrological Guide to Deck, Duels and more

Nightmare Mansion: Echoes of The Abyss

**Nightmare Mansion 2: Legacy of Shadows**

**Nightmare Mansion 3: Shadows of the Forgotten**

Nightmare Mansion 4: Echoes of the Damned

The Life and Banishment of Apophis: Book 2

Nightmare Mansion: Halls of Despair

Healing with Herb: Cannabis and Hydrocephalus

**Planetary Pot: Aligning with Astrological Herbs: Volume 1**

**Fast Track to Freedom: 30 Days to Financial Independence Using AI, Assets, and Agile Hustles**

**Cosmic Hemp Pathways**

**How to Become Financially Free in 30 Days: 10,000 Paths to Prosperity**

**Zodiacal Herbage: Astrological Insights: Volume 1**

Nightmare Mansion: Whispers in the Walls

The Daleks Invade Atlantis

**Henry the hemp and Hydrocephalus**


10X The Kidney Friendly Diet

Cannabis Universe: Adult coloring book

**Hemp Astrology: The Healing Power of the Stars**

**Zodiacal Herbage: Astrological Insights: Cannabis Universe: Volume 2**

<u>**Planetary Pot: Aligning with Astrological Herbs: Cannabis Universes: Volume 2**</u>

Doctor Who Meets the Replicators and SG-1: The Ultimate Battle for Survival

Nightmare Mansion: Curse of the Blood Moon

<u>**The Celestial Stoner: A Guide to the Zodiac**</u>

**Cosmic Pleasures: Sex Toy Astrology for Every Sign**

Hydrocephalus Astrology: Navigating the Stars and Healing Waters

**Lapis and the Mischievous Chocolate Bar**


Celestial Positions: Sexual Astrology for Every Sign

Apophis's Shadow Work Journal: : A Journey of Self-Discovery and Healing

**Kinky Cosmos: Sexual Kink Astrology for Every Sign**

**Digital Cosmos: The Astrological Digimon Compendium**

**Stellar Seeds: The Cosmic Guide to Growing with Astrology**

Apophis's Daily Gratitude Journal


Cat Astrology: Feline Mysteries of the Cosmos

**The Cosmic Kama Sutra: An Astrological Guide to Sexual Positions**

**Unleash Your Potential: A Guided Journal Powered by AI Insights**

**Whispers of the Enchanted Grove**


Cosmic Pleasures: An Astrological Guide to Sexual Kinks

369, 12 Manifestation Journal

Whisper of the nocturne journal(blank journal for writing or drawing)

The Boogey Book

Locked In Reflection: A Chastity Journey Through Locktober
Generating Wealth Quickly:
How to Generate $100,000 in 24 Hours
Star Magic: Harness the Power of the Universe

If you want solar for your home go here: https://www.harborso-lar.live/apophisenterprises/

Get Some Tarot cards: https://www.makeplayingcards.com/sell/apophis-occult-shop

**Get some shirts: https://www.bonfire.com/store/apophis-shirt-emporium/**

<u>**Instagrams:**</u>
@apophis_enterprises,
@apophisbookemporium,
@apophisscardshop
Twitter: @apophisenterpr1
 Tiktok:@apophisenterprise
Youtube: @sg1fan23477, @FiresideRetreatKingdom

**Podcast: Apophis Chat Zone:** https://open.spotify.com/show/
5zXbrCLEV2xzCp8ybrfHsk?si=fb4d4fdbdce44dec

**Newsletter:** https://apophiss-newsletter-27c897.beehiiv.com/